Getting Fit After Fifty

A Complete Guide to Fitness for Men Over 50

Susan D. Rollins

Disclosure Statement

Please be aware that the material in this publication is only intended for educational purposes. Every attempt has been made to offer accurate, current, trustworthy, and comprehensive information. Readers understand that the author is not giving out

professional or medical advice. This book's information came from a variety of sources.

Table of Contents

Chapter 1: The Importance of Fitness for Aging Men

Aging is a natural part of life, but it may come with some unwanted changes, including a decline in physical fitness. Men over the age of 50 may confront several health challenges, from declining muscle mass and bone density to an increased risk of heart disease, diabetes, and other chronic diseases. However, data shows that regular exercise and a healthy lifestyle may help minimize these risks and promote overall health and well-being.

One of the most prominent benefits of exercising for elderly men is greater cardiovascular health.
Cardiovascular activities, such as running, cycling, or swimming, may help lower blood

pressure, reduce the risk of heart disease, and boost overall endurance.

Exercise may also help maintain a healthy weight, which is crucial for decreasing the risk of diabetes, heart disease, and other chronic conditions. Another crucial element of fitness for older men is keeping muscle mass and strength. As men age, they tend to lose muscle mass and bone density, which may lead to fragility and an increased risk of falls and fractures.

However, strength training activities, such as lifting weights or doing bodyweight exercises, may help maintain or even enhance muscle mass and bone density, resulting in higher overall physical function.

In addition to physical health benefits, exercise may also have a good effect on mental health. Regular exercise has been proven to decrease stress, anxiety, and depression, as well as boost cognitive function and overall mood.

Exercise may also be a social activity, which may help overcome loneliness and isolation, a serious concern for older individuals. It's vital to realize that starting a new fitness program could be intimidating, especially for folks who may not have exercised regularly in the past.

However, it's never too late to start. It's crucial to start cautiously and contact a doctor if you have any concerns about your health or any pre-existing difficulties. A combination of aerobic activity, strength training, and flexibility exercises may aid maintain general fitness and minimize the chance of chronic diseases.

In conclusion, exercise and fitness are vital for older men who seek to retain their health and well-being. Exercise may help lessen the risk of chronic diseases, enhance physical function, and promote mental wellness.

It's never too late to start incorporating regular exercise and excellent habits into your daily routine.

Chapter 2: Assessing Your Current Fitness Level

Assessing your current fitness level is a vital step toward improving your health and well-being. By assessing where you are in terms of cardiovascular fitness, strength, flexibility, and balance, you can establish realistic objectives and design a tailored fitness plan that meets your requirements and skills.

Cardiovascular Fitness Assessment

Cardiovascular health refers to your body's potential to switch oxygen for your muscle mass all through activity. A robust cardiovascular system may help minimize your risk of heart disease, stroke, and other chronic illnesses. Measuring your resting heart rate may offer you a general estimate of your cardiovascular fitness level.

A lower resting heart rate is a sign of a stronger cardiovascular system.

Another technique to check your cardiovascular fitness is exercise testing, such as the 1.5-mile run or the step test.

These tests determine how soon your heart rate returns to normal following activity. If your heart rate recovers rapidly, it's an indicator that your circulatory system is powerful.

Strength Assessment

Strength is vital for preserving physical function and minimizing the incidence of falls and fractures. Assessing your strength may be done by workouts such as push-ups, sit-ups, or weightlifting. Count how many repetitions you can do in a given length of time, or pick a weight that is hard but enables you to finish 8 to 12 repetitions.

You may also use a grip strength dynamometer to assess your grip strength. Grip energy is a great degree of ordinary energy and health. A stronger grasp may also assist lower the chances of a disability and untimely mortality.

Flexibility Assessment

Flexibility refers to your body's capacity to move across a complete range of motion. Maintaining flexibility may help minimize the chance of injury and enhance overall physical function. Assessing your flexibility may be done via basic stretches such as the sit-and-reach test. Sit on the floor with your legs straight in front of you and extend forward as far as you can. Measure how far you can reach without straining.

Balance Assessment

Maintaining balance is critical for lowering the risk of falls, particularly as you age. Assessing your balance may be done via activities such as standing on one foot or walking heel-to-toe. Time how long you can stand on one foot or count how many steps you can walk without losing balance.

Once you've analyzed your current fitness level, it's crucial to establish realistic objectives for growth. Consider what areas of fitness you wish to improve and how much time you're prepared to spend exercising each week. It's advised that people obtain at least 150 minutes of moderate-intensity activity or 75 minutes of vigorous-intensity exercise each week, coupled with muscle-strengthening exercises at least two days a week.

Remember to start cautiously and advance gradually. Overexertion or attempting to achieve too much too fast may lead to injury and setbacks. Consulting with a doctor or a competent fitness expert may also be useful, particularly if you have any pre-existing illnesses or worries about your health.

In conclusion, analyzing your current fitness level is a key first step toward improving your health and well-being. By knowing your strengths and areas for growth, you may build a tailored fitness plan that meets your requirements and skills, leading to greater overall physical function and a lower risk of chronic illnesses.

Chapter 3: Designing a Fitness Program for Men Over 50

Designing a fitness program that is suited to your requirements and objectives is crucial to making progress and obtaining results. In this chapter, we'll explore the many components of a well-rounded fitness program for men over 50, including aerobic activity, strength training, flexibility training, and balance training.

Cardiovascular Exercise

Cardiovascular exercise, often known as aerobic exercise, is any activity that boosts your heart rate and breathing rate. This sort of exercise helps increase cardiovascular fitness, lowering the risk of chronic illnesses, and keeping a healthy weight.

For males over 50, it's suggested to strive for at least 150 minutes of moderate-intensity cardio each week, such as brisk walking, cycling, swimming, or dancing.

When establishing a cardiovascular workout program, it's crucial to pick activities that you love and that are suitable for your fitness level. Start with shorter periods and lower intensities, then progressively increase the length and intensity over time. To minimize injury and overuse, it's also crucial to incorporate rest and recovery times in your routine.

Strength Training

Strength training, often known as resistance training, includes utilizing weights or resistance bands to improve your muscles.

This form of exercise is vital for preserving muscle mass, enhancing bone density, and minimizing the risk of age-related muscle loss.

For males over 50, it's suggested to strive for at least two days of strength exercise each week, addressing all main muscle groups.

When establishing a strength training program, it's vital to pick exercises that target particular muscle groups and that are suitable for your fitness level. Start with lighter weights and greater repetitions, then gradually raise the weight and reduce the repetitions over time. It's also crucial to allow for rest and recuperation times in between strength training sessions.

Flexibility Training

Flexibility training includes stretching and moving your muscles and joints to enhance your range of motion and lessen the chance of injury. This form of exercise is crucial for maintaining flexibility, balance, and coordination.

For males over 50, it's suggested to strive for at least two days of flexibility training each week, encompassing stretching exercises for all main muscle groups.

When constructing a flexibility training program, it's vital to pick stretching activities that target particular muscle groups and that are suitable for your fitness level. Start with mild stretches and progressively increase the length and intensity over time.

It's also vital to stretch after various sorts of exercise to help avoid muscular discomfort and damage.

Balance Training

Balance training incorporates activities that stress your balance and coordination to enhance stability and lessen the chance of falls. This form of exercise is especially beneficial for men over 50, who may face decreases in balance and coordination as they age.

For males over 50, it's suggested to strive for at least two days of balance training each week, integrating activities such as standing on one foot, walking heel-to-toe, or practicing yoga or tai chi.

When constructing a balance training program, it's crucial to pick activities that test your balance and coordination but are also acceptable for your fitness level. Start with simpler exercises and progressively move to harder ones over time. It's also crucial to perform balancing exercises in a safe and controlled setting, such as holding onto a sturdy surface or having a spotter nearby.

In conclusion, developing a fitness program that involves aerobic activity, strength training, flexibility training, and balance training is necessary for men over 50 to maintain their overall health and fitness.

By beginning gently, gradually increasing the intensity and length of each form of exercise, and allowing for rest and recovery intervals, men over 50 may develop a fitness program that is personalized to their requirements and objectives and helps them reach maximum health and well-being.

Chapter 4: Strength Training for Men Over 50

Strength training is an important component of a well-rounded fitness program for men over 50. It may help preserve muscle mass, boost bone density, and improve general physical function. In this chapter, we'll cover the advantages of strength training for men over 50 and outline how to get started.

Benefits of Strength Training

Strength training offers various advantages for men over 50, including:

Maintaining muscle mass: As men age, they gradually lose muscle mass, which may contribute to diminished strength and mobility. Strength training may assist maintain muscle mass and prevent muscle atrophy.

Increasing bone density: Strength training may help improve bone density, lowering the incidence of fractures and osteoporosis.

Improving physical function: Strength training may improve balance, coordination, and general physical function, making everyday tasks simpler and minimizing the risk of falls.

Boosting metabolism: Strength training may boost metabolism, helping you burn more calories even at rest.

Improving mental health: Strength training has been demonstrated to boost mood and lessen symptoms of sadness and anxiety.

Getting Started with Strength Training

If you're new to strength training, it's vital to start softly and progressively build intensity and weight over time.

Here are some pointers to get started:

Speak with your healthcare provider: Before beginning any new workout program, it's crucial to speak with your healthcare provider to confirm it's safe for you to do so.

Start with bodyweight exercises: Bodyweight exercises, like squats, push-ups, and lunges, are a fantastic method to increase strength and improve mobility without the need for equipment.

Incorporate resistance training: Resistance exercises, such as using dumbbells or resistance bands, may help grow muscle and boost strength. Start with lesser weights and progressively increase over time.

Focus on form: Proper form is crucial to avoid injury and achieve maximum benefit from strength training activities. Seek help from a licensed personal trainer or fitness expert if required.

Allow for proper rest and recovery: Rest and recovery are necessary for muscle development and injury prevention. Allow for at least one day of recuperation between strength training sessions.

Sample Strength Training Program

Here is a typical strength training regimen for males over 50:

Warm-up: 5-10 minutes of easy cardio, such as walking or cycling, to boost heart rate and prepare the body for activity.

Squats: 2 sets of 10-12 repetitions, using body weight or small weights.

Lunges: 2 sets of 10-12 repetitions, using body weight or light weights.

Push-ups: 2 sets of 10-12 repetitions, altering as required.

Rows: 2 sets of 10-12 repetitions, using dumbbells or resistance bands.

Plank: 2 sets of 30-60 seconds, keeping good form.

Cool-down: 5-10 minutes of stretching to promote flexibility and minimize muscular pain.

In conclusion, strength training is a vital component of a well-rounded fitness program for men over 50. It may help preserve muscle mass, promote bone density, improve physical function, stimulate metabolism, and improve mental wellness. By beginning gently, concentrating on technique, and allowing for proper rest and recovery, men over 50 may safely and efficiently add strength training into their exercise program.

Chapter 5: Cardiovascular Exercise for Men Over 50

Cardiovascular activity is a critical component of maintaining health and fitness, especially for men over 50. In this chapter, we'll explain the advantages of cardiovascular exercise, as well as give practical advice for integrating it into your workout program.

Benefits of Cardiovascular Exercise

Cardiovascular exercise, often known as aerobic exercise, is any activity that boosts your heart rate and breathing rate.

There are various advantages of cardiovascular exercise, including:

Improving heart health: Cardiovascular activity strengthens the heart and enhances its capacity to pump blood throughout the body.

Reducing the risk of chronic illnesses: Cardiovascular exercise may help decrease blood pressure, improve cholesterol levels, and reduce the risk of chronic diseases such as heart disease, diabetes, and some forms of cancer.

Maintaining a healthy weight: Cardiovascular activity burns calories and may help you maintain a healthy weight.

Improving mental health: Cardiovascular activity produces endorphins, which may boost mood and lower the risk of sadness and anxiety.

Types of Cardiovascular Exercise
There are several forms of cardiovascular exercise, including:

Walking: Walking is a low-impact type of cardiovascular exercise that may be done inside or outdoors.

Running: Running is a high-impact kind of cardiovascular exercise that may assist improve cardiovascular fitness and burn calories.

Cycling: Cycling is a low-impact type of cardiovascular exercise that may be done outdoors or on a stationary cycle.

Swimming: Swimming is a low-impact type of cardiovascular exercise that may be good for persons with joint discomfort or injuries.

Group fitness classes: Group fitness programs such as aerobics, Zumba, and dance classes may give a pleasant and sociable method to acquire cardiovascular exercise.

Practical Tips for Incorporating Cardiovascular Exercise

Incorporating cardiovascular activity into your fitness program may be easy and pleasant.

Here are some practical tips:

Start slow: If you're new to cardiovascular fitness, start with a low-impact activity such as walking or cycling and gradually increase the intensity and length of your exercises.

Find activities you enjoy: Choose activities that you find fun and that match your lifestyle. If you don't love jogging, consider swimming or dancing instead.

Mix things up: Incorporate a range of cardiovascular exercises into your regimen to keep it interesting and minimize monotony.

Set reasonable goals: Set reasonable objectives for yourself, such as exercising for 30 minutes a day, three times a week.

Consult with a healthcare provider: If you have any medical ailments or concerns, contact a healthcare physician before beginning a new fitness regimen.

In conclusion, cardiovascular activity is a crucial component of sustaining health and fitness for males over 50. By integrating low-impact activities such as walking or cycling, attempting new activities such as swimming or group exercise courses, and establishing reasonable objectives, men over 50 may improve cardiovascular health, maintain a healthy weight, and minimize the risk of chronic illnesses.

It's crucial to work with a healthcare physician or fitness expert to build a customized exercise regimen that is suited to their unique requirements and objectives.

Chapter 6: Flexibility and Balance Training for Men Over 50

Flexibility and balance training are key components of a well-rounded fitness program, especially for men over 50. In this chapter, we'll explain the advantages of flexibility and balance training, as well as give practical advice for implementing it into your exercise program.

Benefits of Flexibility and Balance Training

Flexibility and balance exercises are vital for maintaining mobility, stability, and general health. As we age, our muscles and joints become less flexible and our balance might become disturbed, which can lead to falls and accidents.

Here are some advantages of flexibility and balance training:

Improving flexibility: Flexibility exercise may enhance the range of motion and joint mobility, minimizing the risk of injury and boosting overall physical performance.

Reducing the risk of falls: Balance training may enhance stability and decrease the risk of falls, which can be especially useful for older persons.

Enhancing physical performance: Flexibility and balance training may boost physical performance and lessen the risk of injury during other types of exercise.

Reducing stress: Flexibility training may assist decrease tension and improve relaxation.

Types of Flexibility and Balance Training
There are several forms of flexibility and balance training, including:
Stretching: Stretching is a sort of flexibility exercise that includes stretching and elongating the muscles to enhance the range of motion and flexibility.

Yoga: Yoga is a kind of flexibility exercise that incorporates stretching, breathing, and relaxing methods to enhance flexibility, balance, and general physical and mental health.

Pilates: Pilates is a style of exercise that focuses on strengthening the core muscles, improving posture, and promoting flexibility and balance.

Tai chi: Tai chi is a sort of low-impact exercise that includes slow, flowing motions and deep breathing to promote balance, flexibility, and general physical and mental health.

Practical Tips for Incorporating Flexibility and Balance Training

Incorporating flexibility and balance training into your exercise program may be straightforward and pleasant.

Here are some practical tips:

Start slow: If you're new to flexibility and balance training, start with easy exercises and progressively increase the intensity and length of your workouts.

Find activities you enjoy: Choose activities that you find fun and that match your lifestyle. If you don't love yoga, try Pilates or Tai Chi instead.

Mix things up: Incorporate a range of flexibility and balancing routines into your regimen to keep it interesting and minimize monotony.

Set reasonable goals: Set reasonable objectives for yourself, such as practicing yoga or Pilates twice a week or attending a Tai Chi session once a week.

Consult with a healthcare provider: If you have any medical ailments or concerns, contact a healthcare physician before beginning a new fitness regimen.

In conclusion, flexibility and balance exercise are crucial components of preserving health and fitness for men over 50. By including stretching, yoga, Pilates, Tai Chi, or other flexibility and balance exercises into their workout regimen, men over 50 may enhance mobility, stability, and physical performance, and minimize the risk of falls and injuries.

It's crucial to work with a healthcare physician or fitness expert to build a customized exercise regimen that is suited to their unique requirements and objectives.

Chapter 7: Nutrition for Men Over 50

As men grow older, their dietary demands shift. In this chapter, we'll cover the special nutritional demands of men over 50 and teach how to make good food choices to promote maximum health and well-being.

Macronutrients

Macronutrients are the nutrients that give energy and are needed in significant quantities in the diet. They comprise carbs, proteins, and lipids. As men age, their bodies may need less energy, but they still require proper quantities of macronutrients to maintain their health.

Carbohydrates are a vital source of energy for the body. Men over 50 should attempt to eat complex carbs, such as whole grains, fruits, and vegetables, rather than simple carbohydrates, such as sugar and processed meals.

Proteins are vital for developing and mending muscular tissue, keeping a healthy immune system, and supporting several other body activities. Men over 50 should attempt to eat lean sources of protein, such as chicken, fish, beans, and tofu.

Fats are crucial for generating energy, stimulating cell development, and protecting organs. Men over 50 should seek to eat healthy fats, such as those found in nuts, seeds, avocados, and fatty fish while minimizing the consumption of saturated and trans fats found in processed foods and animal products.

Micronutrients

Micronutrients are the nutrients necessary in lower quantities in the diet, including vitamins and minerals. As men age, their bodies may need various levels of micronutrients to maintain optimum health.

Calcium is vital for keeping healthy bones and minimizing the incidence of osteoporosis. Men over 50 should attempt to eat enough levels of calcium, found in dairy products, leafy green vegetables, and fortified meals.

Vitamin D is vital for calcium absorption and bone health. Men over 50 should attempt to eat enough quantities of vitamin D, found in fatty fish, egg yolks, and fortified foods, or consider taking a supplement if their levels are low.

B vitamins are crucial for energy generation and sustaining healthy neurons and blood cells. Men over 50 should attempt to take enough levels of B vitamins, found in whole grains, lean meats, and leafy green vegetables.

Hydration

Staying hydrated is vital for maintaining good health, especially as men age. Men over 50 should attempt to consume enough quantities of water throughout the day and restrict the consumption of sugary beverages and alcohol.

Making Healthy Choices

In addition to concentrating on certain macronutrients and micronutrients, men over 50 should also adopt appropriate dietary choices, such as:

Eating a variety of fruits and vegetables to ensure a range of nutrients are taken.

Limiting consumption of processed and high-fat meals.

Eating slowly and carefully enhances digestion and minimizes overeating.

Being aware of portion proportions to provide appropriate but not excessive calorie consumption.

Seeking help from a certified dietician or healthcare practitioner if required.

In conclusion, keeping a balanced diet is vital for men over 50 to preserve their overall health and fitness. By concentrating on particular macronutrients and micronutrients, keeping hydrated, and making appropriate food choices, men over 50 may ensure they are obtaining the nutrients they need to promote optimum health and well-being.

Chapter 8: Mental Health and Well-Being for Men Over 50

Men over 50 tend to disregard their mental health and well-being, even though they are important aspects of total health. In this chapter, we'll talk about the value of mental health and well-being for men over 50 and provide advice on how to keep them in tip-top shape.

The significance of mental health

A person's emotional, psychological, and social well-being are all referred to as mental health. Men over 50 should prioritize their mental health for several reasons, including:

Chronic illness risk is decreased: Chronic disorders including diabetes, heart disease, and stroke are more likely to develop in those who have poor mental health.

Cognitive function may be enhanced and the risk of cognitive decline can be decreased when one has good mental health.

Improved quality of life: Possessing good mental health helps raise life satisfaction and quality of life.

Common Issues with Mental Health

Men over 50 may face several typical mental health issues, such as:

Depression and anxiety: are typical mental health issues in males over the age of 50, and they may significantly reduce the quality of life.

Misuse of substances: Men over 50 who have a history of alcohol or drug use may struggle with substance misuse.

Social isolation: is an issue that many men over 50 experience, and it may be detrimental to mental health.

Techniques for Preserving Mental Health

For men over 50, maintaining excellent mental health is crucial. Some methods for preserving mental health include:

Being active: Regular exercise may enhance mood and lower the chances of anxiety and sadness.

Keeping in touch with friends and family may help lower the risk of social isolation and enhance general mental health.

Getting adequate sleep: Sleep is crucial for maintaining excellent mental and physical health.

Controlling stress: Deep breathing, meditation, and yoga are relaxation methods that may help manage stress and lower the risk of developing depression and anxiety.

Help needed: Maintaining good mental health requires seeking professional assistance if one exhibits signs of depression, anxiety, or other mental health issues.

Conclusion

For males over 50 to preserve total health and well-being, good mental health is crucial. Men over 50 may make sure they are taking care of their mental health by maintaining social relationships, being active, getting adequate sleep, managing stress, and receiving assistance when necessary.

It's crucial to keep in mind that mental health issues are widespread and curable and that asking for assistance is a show of strength.

Chapter 9: Staying Motivated for Fitness as a Man Over 50

At any age, maintaining exercise motivation may be tough, but for men over 50, it can be particularly demanding. We'll talk about methods for maintaining motivation and dedication to fitness in this chapter, as well as how to get through typical roadblocks.

Set attainable objectives

Setting attainable objectives is crucial to maintaining exercise motivation. It's OK for older guys to have different fitness objectives than younger ones. Setting attainable, realistic objectives helps keep you motivated and helps you see results, such as boosting flexibility or strength.

Establish a Routine

Another strategy to maintain your motivation for exercise is to establish a regimen. A regimen may be established by identifying the optimal time of day to exercise and adhering to it. To avoid monotony and keep things fresh, it's also crucial to vary your routines.

Find a Supportive Network

Having a support system might aid in maintaining exercise motivation. Finding a personal trainer, joining a fitness program, or working out with a buddy may provide accountability and motivation.

Overcoming Challenges

When it comes to fitness, men over 50 may have special challenges, such as physical restrictions or time restraints.

Finding solutions to these challenges, such as modifying exercises to account for physical restrictions or figuring out how to fit exercise into everyday schedules, will help you remain on track.

Promote Progress

Celebrating accomplishments is a crucial component of maintaining fitness motivation. Noticing advancements, such as greater strength or endurance, might inspire one to keep continuing by giving one a feeling of success.

Conclusion

Men over 50 may maintain their commitment to their exercise objectives by establishing reasonable goals, developing a regimen, finding a support system, conquering challenges, and recognizing accomplishment. Keep in mind that improving your fitness takes time and is a process. Men over 50 may reach their exercise objectives and keep up their best health and well-being by being regular and devoted.